VShred Endomorph Diet Plan

7-Step proven Approach to Unlock Your Body's Potential: Effective Strategies for Fat Loss, Muscle Gain, and Improved Health

MEGAN

REWARD

Take Your Endomorph Journey to the Next Level!

Dear Reader,

I know how challenging it can be to stay on track with your ***diet, fitness, and weight loss goals*** as an endomorph. After receiving countless requests and fueled by my passion to truly help you succeed, I've created something special—an ***All-in-One Endomorph Diet & Fitness Tracker!***

This ***70-page tracking template*** is designed *to* ***simplify your journey, keep you accountable, and help you track progress effortlessly***—from meal planning and calorie tracking to workout logs and habit-building sections.

Scan the QR code or follow the link below to get instant access to your Endomorph Diet & Fitness Tracker!

https://megan-publishing.kit.com/874653decd

MEGAN

Table of Contents

Your Roadmap to Success: Track, Plan, and Achieve!

Success in your health and fitness journey isn't just about knowing what to do—it's about staying consistent and making steady progress. That's why I've included Endomorph Diet Planning and Fitness Tracking Templates to help turn knowledge into action.

With these templates, you'll be able to:

☑ Plan meals that support fat loss and muscle growth.

☑ Track your workouts to stay motivated and measure improvements.

☑ Monitor your progress so you can adjust and refine your approach.

When you track your habits, you stay accountable—and when you stay accountable, you see results. These templates are your personal guide to making your diet and fitness routine work for you.

Find them below, start using them today, and take charge of your transformation!

Templates list for this book.

- Note Template
- 90 Days Body Goal Template
- 30 Days Challenge Template

- My Daily Fitness Template
- Sleep Tracker Template
- Workout Log Template
- Favorite Food Tracker Template
- Food Tracker Template
- Weekly Workout Tracker Template
- Weekly Meal Planner Template
- Habits Tracker Template
- Weekly Measurement Tracker

INTRODUCTION

Understand Your Body Type: Endomorph

Body types are important in fitness and nutrition because they outline the optimal meals and exercise routines. The endomorph is distinguished from the other two major body types, the mesomorph and the ectomorph, by its distinct traits and problems. If you're reading this, you probably identify as an endomorph or want to learn more about this body type.

Endomorphs are typically softer and rounder in shape, with a larger waist, stronger bone structure, and a tendency to gain weight faster than other body types. An endomorph's metabolism is typically slower, making weight loss appear difficult. When confronted with excessive expectations imposed by the fitness industry and the media, it is easy to become frustrated and discouraged.

However, it is crucial to remember that being an endomorph is simply a different starting place on the journey to fitness and health, not a limitation. Accepting your body type may increase your confidence and ability to make needs-based decisions. Endomorphs can increase their general health and muscular growth while losing weight if they have the proper knowledge and procedures.

Determining your body type is the first step toward realizing your full potential. The VShred Endomorph Diet Plan was designed specifically to meet endomorph needs. To help people achieve long-term success, it addresses the specific difficulties they face and offers approaches that are both effective and scientifically supported.

The Scientific Basis for the Methodology: How This Diet Works

The VShred Endomorph Diet Plan is based on a thorough understanding of nutrition and metabolism. Unlike diets designed for all body types, this technique is specifically targeted to the needs of endomorphs, allowing you to reach your goals of fat loss, muscle building, and overall health.

According to the study, endomorphs respond better to a diet strong in protein, healthy fats, and carbohydrates. This isn't a passing fad; it's a fundamental aspect of how our bodies absorb food. Protein is essential for endomorphs looking to bulk up their bodies since it supports muscle growth and repair. Good fats are needed for hormone synthesis and overall health, whereas managed carbohydrate consumption promotes fat loss and maintains insulin levels.

Furthermore, the timing of nutrients and the calorie balance are key components of this diet. Understanding how to plan your meals and alter your calorie intake based on your activity level will help your body burn fat rather than store it. Unlike typical diets, the VShred Endomorph Diet adopts a more nuanced approach, accounting for the significant variances between body types.

The evidence is clear: supplying your body with the proper nutrients in the right amounts will help you function optimally and get the best results. The VShred Endomorph Diet Plan builds a success roadmap on this scientific foundation, allowing you to take charge of your health and attain the body you want.

Tips to Make the Most of This Book

It is critical that you utilize this book as your personal road map and guide while embarking on this journey. The VShred Endomorph Diet Plan aims to equip you with thorough knowledge and realistic techniques for reaching your body's full potential. Here's how to get the most out of what's within

Read With Intention: Give each chapter your full attention. Understanding the fundamental ideas will improve your overall experience and outcomes, as the knowledge supplied is intended to be built upon. Before beginning any diet or exercise regimens, perform an honest assessment of yourself to gain a better understanding of your present habits, lifestyle, and aspirations. This book includes contemplation exercises and questions to help you determine where you are and where you want to go.

Set Reasonable Goals: The primary goal of this trip is to make progress rather than perfection. Set realistic short- and long-term goals based on your tastes and lifestyle. Reward yourself for tiny accomplishments along the way to keep your motivation up.

Engage with the Content: Take notes, highlight significant topics, and consider how they apply to your own circumstance. Do not simply read the text without considering. Engaging in the exercise will motivate you to take action and reinforce the ideas you've learnt.

Plan and Prepare: Using the meal planning and preparation ideas in this book, create a schedule that works for you. Meal planning is vital for endomorphs since it keeps them on track and prevents impulsive eating.

Put the Strategies to Work by Taking Action! The main value of this book is in its applications. To achieve the desired outcomes, adhere to a thorough diet, exercise program, and mental health measures.

Keep your attention and adaptability in mind: this is a marathon, not a sprint. It's crucial to stick to your plan, but you should also be willing to change your strategy along the road. Pay attention to your measurements and make adjustments as needed to ensure continual progress.

Interact with the Community: Consider joining online or local organizations where you can share your experiences, ask questions, and receive assistance. Being surrounded by others who share your values will greatly increase your motivation and productivity.

Following these guidelines will set you up for a successful trip to weight loss, muscle building, and increased health. The VShred Endomorph Diet Plan allows you to attain your highest potential and live your best life. It extends beyond merely a diet.

As you read this book, keep in mind that each step you take brings you closer to your goals. Have faith in science, believe in yourself, and understand that the process is vital for success. This is the beginning of your journey to improve your life and physique.

(Chapter 1:)

Seven Simple Steps to Reach Your Full Potential.

It might be intimidating to start a journey towards health and fitness, especially for those of us who lean andromorphically. However, if you utilize the appropriate tactics and have the right attitude, you may achieve your goals and maximize your physical talents. This chapter describes a simple seven-step technique created exclusively for endomorphs. Understanding your own body type, setting realistic goals, mastering nutrition, and combining beneficial activities can lay the groundwork for long-term success.

Journey to Full Potential

Positive Mindset
Implement Diet
kJ
Exercise Plans
Meal Preparation
Dietary Practices
Set Objectives
Evaluate Body Type

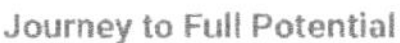

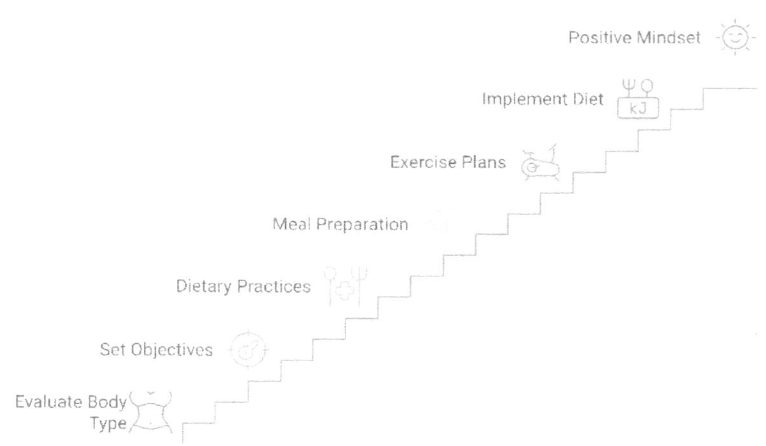

1. Evaluate Your Body Type

properties of endomorphs

Before getting into the intricacies of nutrition and exercise, it's vital to define what it means to be an endomorph. Endomorphs typically exhibit the following traits:

Endomorphs tend to have larger hips and waists and are naturally curvaceous.
Simpler Fat accumulate: People with this body type are more likely to accumulate weight, particularly around their midsection.

Stronger Lower Body: Endomorphs are excellent lower body strength trainers since they typically have strong legs.

Slower Metabolism: Because endomorphs have a slower metabolic rate than other body types, they may struggle to lose weight.

Knowing these characteristics allows you to adjust your approach to better reflect your natural tendencies. Remember that being an endomorph might be beneficial rather than detrimental if you have the proper information.

Test of Self-Evaluation

To learn more about your body type and how it affects your fitness journey, fill out this self-assessment quiz. Give a real response to every inquiry:

What body type are you?

a) Slim and trim.

b) Well-built and durable

c) Round and flexible.

How quickly do you gain weight?

a) Firmly.

b) Lightly.

c) Very easy.

Where do you usually keep extra fat?

a) Especially in the arms and legs.

b) distributed evenly.

c) Around the waist and hips.

How would you describe your metabolic process?

a) Swift

b) Average.

c) Lethargic.

How do you feel about strength training.

a) It's not one of my favorites, however.

b) I enjoy it.

c) I am quite skilled at it.

Score:

Most A's: You might not be an endomorph.

Most of the BS: You could be a mesomorph.

Most c's: You most likely identify as an endomorph.

This self-assessment defines your body type, laying the framework for the subsequent actions. To maximize your potential, you must first have an understanding of yourself.

2. Having reasonable objectives.

Goals: Immediate versus Extended

Goals are necessary for any fitness program, but endomorphs must strike the correct balance of pragmatism and desire. Let's divide these into short-term and long-term aims.

Short-term goals: are ones that can be accomplished in a few weeks or months. These could include meeting a specific weight loss goal, fitting into a specific size of clothing, or exercising a set number of times per week. Short-term goals are intended to function as motivational anchors, keeping you on track and providing rapid reward.

Long-Term Goals: These are more ambitious and aspirational, and they usually take six months or longer to attain. Long-term goals include achieving a certain weight, running a half-marathon, or gaining significant muscular mass. They necessitate effort, patience, and a carefully planned strategy.

The importance of monitoring development

Tracking your progress is crucial if you want to stay motivated and alter your strategy as needed. Keep track of your food, exercise routine, and feelings about your success in a journal or app. For this reason, observation is critical.

Accountability: Writing down your efforts makes you more accountable to yourself.

Awareness: By researching what works and what does not, you will be able to tailor your approach.

Celebration: Keeping an eye on progress allows you to identify and value tiny successes, which encourages positive behavior.

Before you go, make a plan for your travel that includes both short- and long-term goals, and commit to checking in with yourself on a regular basis to assess how you're doing. This practice will help you stay motivated and focused as you strive to fulfill your potential.

3. Fundamentals of Dietary Practices

Good diet is the foundation of any successful training regimen, particularly for endomorphs. This section will break down the principles of macronutrients, micronutrients, and water to help you create a well-balanced diet that promotes muscle building and fat loss.

What Macronutrients Mean

Macronutrients are nutrients that are required for both development and maintenance while also providing us with energy. Lipids, proteins, and carbohydrates make up the vast majority of them.

Understanding how each affects your diet is critical for endomorphs.

Proteins are the structural components of muscle. As an endomorph, you should aim for a higher protein consumption to aid muscle development and repair. Good sources include eggs, fish, poultry, lean meats, and plant-based proteins such lentils and tofu.

Carbohydrates, while sometimes despised, are necessary for energy, particularly while participating in physical activity. Concentrate on complex carbohydrates, like those found in fruits, vegetables, and whole grains. They give consistent energy and are high in nutrients.

Good fats are essential for hormonal synthesis and overall wellness. Incorporate avocados, almonds, seeds, and olive oil into your meals. Remember that being overweight does not mean being obese; balance and moderation are essential.

Endomorphs should aim for a macronutrient ratio that favors more protein and healthy fats while consuming moderate amounts of carbohydrates. This balance regulates insulin levels, promoting muscle growth and fat elimination.

Value of Small Nutrients

Regardless of how important macronutrients are, micronutrients should not be underestimated. Vitamins and minerals are essential for good health, accelerated metabolism, and improved performance. Eat a variety of colored fruits and vegetables to ensure you're getting enough nutrients. Endomorphs require several micronutrients, including:

Magnesium: promotes energy production and muscle function.

Vitamin D: Required for strong bones and an immune system.

B vitamins: Reduce weariness and aid in energy metabolism.

Hydration's Effect on Health

Water is essential for overall health and weight loss, although being often overlooked. Hydration boosts metabolism, eases digestion, and improves athletic performance. Aim for a daily water intake of half your body weight in ounces, and increase it when you exercise.

Suggestion:

Begin your day with a glass of water and keep yourself hydrated by carrying a reusable water bottle.

4. Organizing and preparing meals

How well you plan and cook your meals can make all the difference in your success. Making it a habit to prepare and plan meals ahead of time can help you succeed.

Create a Weekly Meal Plan

To start each week, make a weekly meal plan. Here's how you can successfully do it:

Choose recipes that meet your macronutrient targets: while still being enjoyable to consume. At each meal, aim for a balanced protein, fat, and carbohydrate intake.

Make a Schedule: Allocate certain days for meal preparation. To ensure that you follow through, mark a time window on your calendar.

Portion Control: Consider how large your serving sizes are. Use measuring cups or food scales to ensure you are consuming the correct amount.

Variety: Use a variety of foods every week to avoid monotony and promote a well-rounded nutritional intake.

savvy tips for supermarket shopping

Grocery shopping might be intimidating, but there are a few clever tactics you can employ to make it go more smoothly:

Make a List: Using your meal plan, create a list of everything you'll need to avoid making impulsive purchases.

Shop the Periphery: Fresh produce, proteins, and dairy products are often available in the supermarket's outer aisles. Pay great attention to the following areas.

Seasonal Produce: Choose fruits and vegetables that are in season for the best flavor and cost savings.

When purchasing packaged items, check the labels carefully and keep an eye out for extra sugars and bad fats.

Effective Techniques for Meal Planning.

Meal planning is your best companion on this journey. Here are a few approaches to simplifying things:

Cooking in bulk: Make a huge batch of veggies, meats, and cereals at once. Divide them up so you can easily access them all week.

Use Containers: Purchase high-quality meal prep containers to store your meals. Clear containers allow you to see exactly what you have on hand.

Freeze Extras: You can save leftover food for later use by freezing it. This minimizes waste and ensures that you always have healthy options on hand.

Developing a meal planning and preparation technique will minimize stress, offer you more time, and make it easier to select healthier options.

5. Excellent Exercise Plans for Endomorphs

Exercise is essential for any weight loss or muscle gain program. Endomorphs must strike the appropriate balance of strength training, cardio, and flexibility to achieve the best results.

Fundamentals of Strength Training

Endomorphs benefit greatly from strength training. Gaining muscle can increase your resting metabolic rate, which can help you lose weight. Here are some guidelines to adhere to:

Stress Compound Movements: Multi-muscle strengthening activities such as bench presses, squats, deadlifts, and rows are quite beneficial.

Lift Weights Frequently: Aim for three to four strength training sessions per week. Changing up your workout routine will help you target different muscles.

Progressive Overload: Gradually add weights or resistance to keep your muscles stretched.

Techniques For Cardiovascular Fat Loss

Furthermore, cardiovascular activity is necessary, especially for improving cardiovascular health and burning calories. Consider the strategies below:

High-intensity interval training (HIIT): is a type of exercise that consists of short bursts of high-intensity activity followed by rest periods, and it may be particularly beneficial for fat loss. Aim to do 20–30-minute HIIT exercises many times each week.

Exercise in a Steady State: Include long periods of moderate-intensity walking, running, or cycling. Aim for 150 minutes of moderate activity per week.

Variate your aerobic routines to keep things interesting. For a change of pace, consider dance, swimming, or group lessons.

Flexibility and Recovery

Never underestimate the importance of recovery and adaptation in your training regimen. Yoga, foam rolling, and stretching can all help you increase your flexibility, heal faster, and avoid injurie

Stretching should always be included in your post-workout cool-down routine.

Rest Days: Take regular breaks to allow your body to recover and replenish. This is critical for long-term success.

Strength training, cardio, and flexibility exercises can work together to create a well-rounded fitness plan that will help you achieve your goals.

6. Putting Diet into Practice

Now that you have the knowledge, it is time to put the diet into action. This section includes helpful advice, sample menus, and snack ideas to help you succeed.

Example of a daily meal plan

To get you started, here is a sample menu:

For Breakfast:

Three scrambled eggs with spinach and tomatoes.

One whole-grain piece of bread.

One tablespoon of avocado.

Snack:

Berries combined with some Greek yogurt and chia seeds.

Lunch:

A grilled chicken breast.
Quinoa salad topped with cucumbers, bell peppers, and olive oil.

Snack:

Dip carrot sticks in hummus.

Dinners:

roasted vegetables on the side, baked salmon
Sweet potatoes mashed

MEGAN

Snack for the evening:

A little handful of almonds or walnuts.

Snack Ideas and Portion Control

Even if it is challenging at times, endomorphs must choose nutritious snacks.

Here are a few recommendations:

Nuts and seeds: are high in healthy fats and protein; however, they should be used in moderation.

Fruits: Instead of drinking fruit juice, consider eating entire fruits to get more fiber and minerals.

Vegetable Sticks: Serve with guacamole or hummus, both healthy dips.

Controlling the size of portions is critical. Use smaller plates, measure portion sizes, and listen to your body's hunger signals.

Modifying Your Nutrition in Response to Advancements

The way your body reacts to the diet will primarily decide how successful you are. Keep an eye on your progress and tweak as needed:

Track Changes: Keep track of your meals and weight reduction with a food journal or app.

Be adaptable: If you reach a plateau, consider changing your training routine, macronutrient ratios, or calorie intake.

Consult an Expert: Consider working with a personal trainer or dietitian who may offer tailored advice based on your specific requirements.

7. Drive and Attitude.

Achieving your goals requires more than just physical improvements; you must also create the proper mentality. This section focuses on building a support network, overcoming mental challenges, and remaining dedicated in the face of adversity.

Overcoming Mental Difficulties.

Mental difficulties can be the greatest impediment to achievement. Common challenges include:

When you doubt yourself, remind yourself of your strengths and accomplishments. Set progress ahead of perfection.

Accept your fear of failure as a learning opportunity. Every difficulty has the potential to lead to growth.

Negative Self-Talk: Replace negative thoughts with words of strength. Motivate yourself as you would a buddy.

Developing a Network of Assistance

Having a strong support network can dramatically increase your drive and success. Here's how you can receive more of that assistance.

Find Accountability Partners: by taking a fitness class, finding a workout partner, or communicating with like-minded people on social media.

Seek Professional guidance: If you want sound guidance and support, speak with a nutritionist or trainer.

Celebrate Together: To retain accountability and motivation, inform your network of supporters about your accomplishments.

Staying Committed in the Face of Difficulties.

Every journey will have its highs and lows. Keeping dedicated when things get rough is key.

Remind Yourself of Your Why: Never forget why you chose this road and what you hope to achieve.

Adapt and Triumph: Take a flexible approach. Never be afraid to try new approaches if something isn't working.

Develop Self-Compassion: Recognize that everyone experiences challenges. Treat yourself with kindness and perseverance.

By following this 7-step method, you put yourself in a good position to reach your body's full potential. This approach involves assessing your body type, setting appropriate goals, mastering nutrition, implementing successful workouts, and developing the right mindset. Accept the challenge, trust in science, and believe in your ability to change your life.

Notes

Notes

(Chapter 2:)

Common Mistakes and Their Avoidance

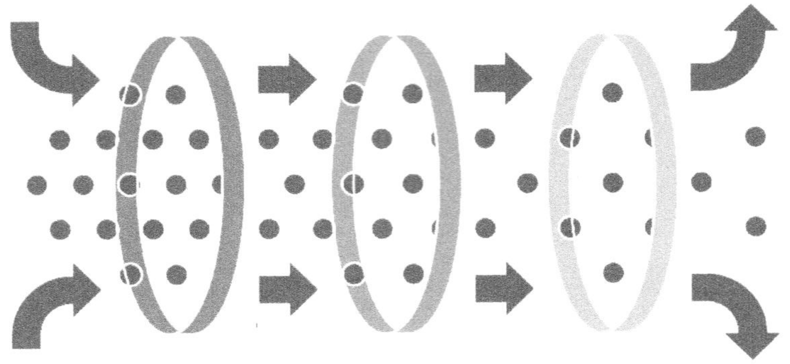

Obstacles will undoubtedly arise in the pursuit of health and fitness. As an endomorph, you may encounter specific hurdles that impede your progress. However, being conscious of these challenges—such as regulating desires, avoiding emotional eating, and remaining consistent—will allow you to successfully navigate your route. In this chapter, we will look at common challenges and provide practical answers.

1. Recognize Emotional Consumption.

Many people suffer emotional eating, which is particularly obvious in endomorphs. Common reasons for this behavior include stress, boredom, sadness, and even celebration. The first step in effectively regulating emotional eating is to identify its causes.

Emotional Eating: What Is It?

Emotional eating occurs when people eat not to satisfy their hunger, but to cope with their emotions. This type of behavior might lead to overeating and make it more difficult to maintain a healthy lifestyle.

The following are some common emotional eating triggers:

Stress: When stressed, people tend to seek comfort meals that are high in sugar or fat.

Boredom: can lead to mindless nibbling and excessive calorie consumption.

Sadness or loneliness: When confronted with emotional distress, some people turn to food for solace; they find comfort in their favorite treats.

Celebration: On the other side, many individuals incorrectly associate food with festivities, which can lead to overindulgence when people gather.

Identifying Causes of Emotional Eating

Knowing what your triggers are is critical for avoiding emotional eating. The following approaches will help you recognize emotional eating.

Keep a food journal in which you record everything you eat: when you consume it, and how you feel right now. Your capacity to identify trends and emotional triggers will increase with experience.

"Why?" is a question you should ask yourself.: Think carefully before reaching for a snack to discover whether you are truly hungry or if there is another reason you are seeking food.

Seek Patterns: You may finally discover specific situations or feelings that cause emotional eating. Identifying these trends is vital for developing more effective coping techniques.

How to Break Free from Emotional Eating

Once you've identified your triggers, it's essential to take steps to manage emotional eating:

Look for Alternative Coping Mechanisms: Look for other ways to deal with emotions outside eating. Consider indulging in hobbies such as journal writing, walking, meditating, or deep breathing exercises.

Practice Mindful Eating: Eat slowly and taste your food. Mindfulness can help you become more aware of your body's cues of hunger and fullness.

Create a Support System: Tell your friends and family about your problems so they can provide you advice and help when you're feeling low.

Taking care of your emotional eating habits will help you keep to your diet and exercise routine.

2. How to Deal with Cravings and Their Significance

Strong and difficult to ignore cravings may emerge, especially when attempting to keep to a diet plan. Your success is dependent on understanding the nature of cravings and implementing effective management tactics.

Understanding cravings

Cravings are intense eating inclinations that are often driven by physiological or emotional factors. The following are some common causes of cravings that you may encounter.

Nutritional Deficiencies: If you are deficient in certain nutrients, your body may seek out certain foods. A chocolate addiction, for example, can indicate a magnesium deficiency.

Hormonal Changes: Cravings for specific foods, especially sweets, may be caused by hormonal shifts, particularly during menstruation.

Psychological Triggers: Stress, boredom, and habit can all serve as triggers for cravings, as well as emotional eating.

Recognize your desires.

Recognizing the nature of cravings is the first step toward overcoming them. Consider asking these questions:

What kind of cuisine do I wish to try? Is it sweet, salty, fatty, or a combination?

When do I usually feel a need for these things? Are they related to specific times of the day, activities, or emotions?

Is this really a craving, or is there anything else going on? You can use this reflection to decide if you should indulge or choose a healthier alternative.

Techniques to Control Cravings

Although cravings are a normal part of life, there are a few ways you may use to effectively suppress them.

Drink plenty of water: as hunger and thirst can be confused. Make sure you have enough water to drink during the day.

Include Healthier Substitutions: If you have a sweet tooth, go for fruit instead of candy. Consider roasted nuts or air-popped popcorn to fulfill your salt cravings.

Exercise Portion Control: If you decide to give in to a craving, do so mindfully. Rather than starving yourself to death, let yourself a small amount. This strategy can help prevent feelings of deprivation, which may contribute to binge eating later.

Distract Yourself: Do everything to take your focus away from food desires when they occur. Distractions, like as going for a walk, calling a friend, or doing something fun, can help to alleviate the severity of cravings.

Understanding and regulating your wants can allow you to stick to your diet without feeling deprived.

3. Staying True to Your Plan

When it comes to achieving your fitness and health goals, consistency is key. However, sticking to a diet and exercise plan can be challenging, especially when barriers or temptations occur. Here are some strategies to help you maintain your consistency.

The Value of Consistency

Establishing a consistent eating and exercise schedule is critical to your long-term success.

MEGAN

Routines can help automate your decision-making, making it easier to stick to your strategy. Here's how to establish a dependable routine:

Create Meal and Exercise Schedules: Try to eat and exercise at the same times each day. Maintaining this constancy allows your body to adapt and keeps you on track.

Allow for Flexibility: Because life is unpredictable, leave some wiggle room in your daily routine. If you have a busy day, prepare your meals ahead of time or choose shorter workouts that will still fit into your schedule.

Overcome Obstacles

Obstacles are unavoidable on any journey; thus, it is vital to keep moving forward in the face of setbacks.

The following are strategies to overcome obstacles:

Do not dwell on your mistakes: If you overeat junk food or ignore your workout routine, accept it guilt-free, learn from it, and move on. Rehashing errors might make you feel horrible about yourself and increase your chances of giving up.

Reevaluate Your Goals: If you are consistently struggling to achieve your objectives, take a step back and reconsider them. Make sure they fit your lifestyle and are affordable.

Evaluate Your Progress: Regularly examine your achievements and advancements. Recognize your accomplishments, no matter how modest, to keep your spirits high and your thinking positive.

Creating A Helpful Environment

Establishing an environment that motivates you to achieve your goals will significantly enhance your consistency. The following tips can help you establish a pleasant environment:

Stock Your Kitchen Wisely: Fill your fridge and cupboard with nutritious, diet-friendly snacks and foods. Eliminate temptations that may obstruct your progress.

Engage Others: Tell your family and friends about your aspirations. Engage them in your journey by sharing meals, exercising together, or having encouraging chats.

Make Reminders: Use visual reminders to help you stay on track with your goals. Put uplifting phrases on your fridge or set phone reminders.

Your success with the endomorph diet plan is dependent on avoiding typical pitfalls like as emotional eating, cravings, and inconsistencies. By becoming aware of your triggers and implementing effective tactics, you will be more equipped to overcome difficulties and stay on track with your goals. Remember that the journey is about more than just reaching to your destination; it's also about enjoying the ride and finding new facets of yourself.

Remember these strategies as you go, and stay adaptable. You have the ability to maximize your body's potential and build the life you want. Let's take this adventure together, one step at a time.

Notes

Notes

(Chapter 3:)

Achievements.

Success is frequently best measured by the experiences of those who have accepted their journeys, conquered challenges, and improved their lives, rather than by numbers on a scale. This chapter will look at actual changes, make crucial inferences from their experiences, and provide useful advice from endomorphs who have succeeded and reached their full potential by following the VShred Endomorph Diet Plan.

I. Actual Life Changes

First Transformation Story: Sarah's Path

Sarah, a 32-year-old graphic designer, has struggled with her weight throughout her adult life. She identified as an endomorph and struggled to lose weight despite numerous diets and exercise regimes. Sarah, feeling deflated and disappointed, decided to try something else.

The Tipping Point

Sarah discovered that the VShred Endomorph Diet Plan was specifically developed for her body type. She started by assessing her body type, setting realistic goals, and focusing equally on fat loss and muscle gain. Sarah vowed to maintain a consistent workout routine that included both high-intensity interval training (HIIT) and strength training. She also learnt how to cook nutritious meals that satisfied her cravings without impeding her progress.

Conclusions

Sarah shed thirty pounds and acquired a lot of strength and vigor in just six months. More significantly, she formed a positive relationship with food and learned to listen to her body's cues. Sarah continues, "It's about feeling strong and empowered; it's not just about losing weight."

Tale of Metamorphosis II: Mark's Adventure

Mark, a 28-year-old software developer, met the normal problems that an endomorph faces. Because of his sedentary employment and fondness of late-night snacking, he suffered with weight gain and low self-esteem. Mark attended the VShred vacation because he wanted to enhance his lifestyle.

The Plan

Mark began by becoming aware of the triggers that cause him to eat emotionally and then practiced mindful eating. He planned nutritious meals using the meal planning skills he learned in class. He also added regular workouts that focused on increasing overload in strength training.

Conclusions

In just four months, Mark transformed not just his physical appearance but also his mind. He had reduced 25 pounds and felt more confident in social situations. I discovered that consistency is essential.

"It's about development, not perfection," Mark adds.

The Third Story of Transformation: Lisa's Climb

Lisa, a 45-year-old endomorph, had been suffering with her weight for years and felt stuck in a cycle of emotional eating and dieting. She often felt hopeless and thought she'd never attain her objectives until she discovered the VShred Endomorph Diet Plan.

The Journey

Lisa's path required a full transformation of her lifestyle. She sought to identify her body type and create achievable goals. She motivated herself by documenting her development and enjoying minor triumphs. Lisa also joined an online support group, which was quite helpful to her.

Conclusions

After a year of hard work, Lisa shed fifty pounds, toned her muscles, and, most importantly, discovered a new passion for cooking and working out. She added with a grin, "I feel like I'm living my best life now." "You can always change your story at any time."

2. Conclusions Drawn from The Event

These motivational makeovers highlight crucial concepts that can benefit anyone aspiring for success:

Lesson 1: embrace your body type.

To adapt your strategy, first recognize and accept your body type. The VShred Endomorph Diet Plan emphasizes nutritious food and effective exercise to fulfill endomorphs' special demands. Understanding your individual physiology allows you to build techniques that are most beneficial for you.

Lesson 2: Set fair and doable objectives.

Achievable goals are essential for maintaining motivation and avoiding feelings of failure. Divide your more difficult goals into manageable milestones. Recognize little victories to boost confidence and momentum.

Lesson 3: Prioritize progress over perfection.

Seeking perfection could lead to dissatisfaction and exhaustion. Instead, concentrate on making gradual gains. Recognize that hurdles are common, and how you navigate them is what matters most.

Lesson 4: Create a Network of Support

A strong support network can have a significant impact on your success. Be in the presence of people who understand your problems and celebrate your triumphs. Engage with online communities, friends, and family members who may offer support and accountability.

Lesson 5: Pay care to your mental health.

Mental health and physical transformation frequently go hand in hand. Journaling, mindfulness, and meditation are all tools that can help you manage stress and emotional eating. Persistent success necessitates optimism.

3. Wisdom from Reaching Endomorphs

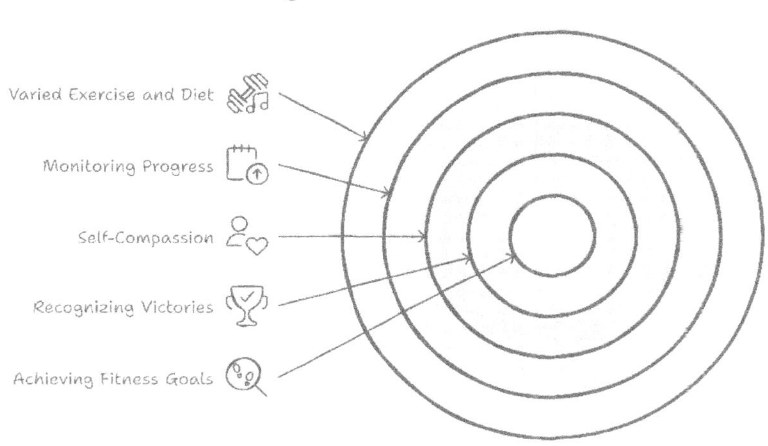

Based on the experiences of successful endomorphs, the following practical advice can aid you along the way:

Tip 1: bit of advice: customize your menu.

Customize your diet to fit your preferences and lifestyle. Experiment with various recipes and meal combinations to determine what works best for you. Eating well is critical for maintaining a long-term diet.

Tip 2: Change up your exercise routines.

Mix strength training, cardio, and flexibility workouts to keep things interesting and your body challenged in new ways. This will lessen boredom while increasing dedication.

Tip 3: Monitor your development.

Keep a notebook or use apps to monitor your nutrition, activity, and progress. Seeing tangible results can be highly motivating and inspire you to stick to your goals.

Tip 4: Show Compassion for Yourself

Be nice to yourself while traveling. Recognize that everyone experiences difficulties and setbacks. Develop self-compassion. Don't let a mistake keep you from moving forward; instead, view it as an opportunity to develop.

Tip 5: Recognize each victory.

Celebrate your achievements, no matter how minor. Whether it's completing a difficult workout, resisting an urge, or losing a size in your wardrobe, noticing and appreciating every small win will keep you motivated.

The inspiring experiences of Sarah, Mark, and Lisa serve as compelling reminders that change is attainable. If you accept their travels, learn from them, and follow some helpful suggestions, you, too, can reach your full potential. After all, each step you take brings you closer to your goal.

Allow these stories to inspire and drive you as you pursue your own goals. Regardless of the barriers in your path, you can achieve the change you desire if you are committed to pushing forward, have support, and are dedicated to your objectives. Let us continue this voyage together, motivated by the belief that achievement is within reach.

Notes

Notes

(Chapter 4:)

Sophisticated Techniques for Continuous Improvement

Regardless of how long you've been a part of the program, there comes a time where fine-tuning your strategies might help you grow even faster. This chapter will go over advanced strategies such as changing your food to achieve different goals, using endomorph-specific supplements, and fine-tuning your exercise regimen for long-term success. Starting the VShred Endomorph Diet Plan has already given you a huge advantage in fulfilling your body's true potential.

1. Nutritional Modifications for Different Goals

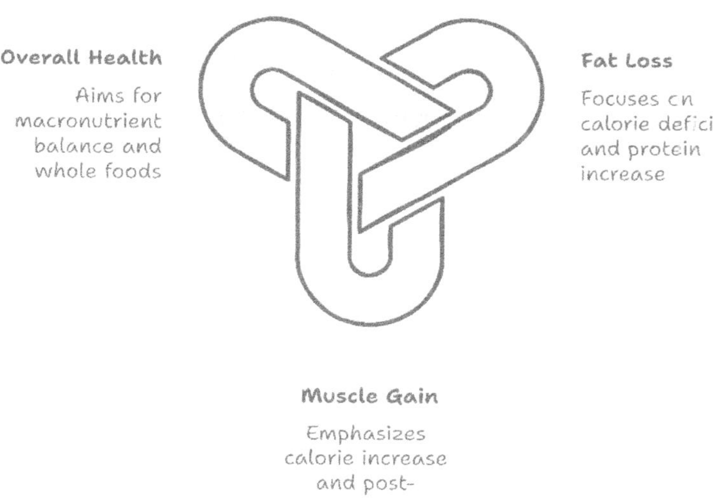

Your nutritional demands will most likely vary as you progress, so you must adapt your diet to meet your new objectives in order to reap the rewards. Whether your aim is to improve your overall health, develop muscle mass, or lose weight, these small changes will get you there faster.

loss of fat

If your primary objective is to reduce weight, you must adhere to your diet plan religiously. However, after a period, your body is likely to react to a calorie deficit, and you may reach a plateau. Small dietary changes can then help you lose fat again.

Key Modifications for Fat Loss:

Slight calorie deficit: As you lose weight, your initial calorie intake may become too high due to decreased metabolic demands. A daily calorie reduction of 100-200 may help you build the deficit needed to break through a plateau.

Carb Cycling: Because carbs are a difficult macronutrient for endomorphs, you can boost fat loss by including carb cycling into your diet. This entails consuming more carbs on training days to boost performance and fewer carbohydrates on recovery days to reduce fat storage.

Increase Your Protein Intake: Increasing your protein intake by ten to fifteen percent will aid in fat loss while preserving lean muscle composition. Protein is not only necessary for muscular growth, but it also has a thermogenic effect, which means that digesting protein expends more calories than burning fat or carbohydrates.

An example of a meal modification to reduce fat.

For dinner, replace the heavy carbs with a high-protein option such as Greek yogurt or cottage cheese topped with berries. To obtain some healthy fats, try grilled chicken salad with mixed vegetables, olive oil, and a handful of nuts.

Increased Muscle

Endomorphs can gain muscle, but it takes a mix of strength training and proper nutrition. When shifting from a fat-loss phase to a muscle-building phase, gradually increase your caloric intake, with a focus on high-quality foods.

Important Changes to Gain Muscle:

Increase Calorie Intake Gradually: When beginning a muscle-building phase, aim for a 5-10% daily increase in calories. Concentrate on lean protein, balanced carbohydrates, and healthy fats.

Consider Your Post-Workout Nutrition: Because muscle growth and recuperation occur in the hours following exercise, it's critical to consume a post-workout meal or smoothie that contains both quickly digesting carbohydrates (such as rice cakes or lean meat) and protein (such as whey protein).

Maximize Carbohydrate Intake Before and After Exercise: Consuming more carbohydrates before and after exercise can help fuel your training and muscle-building efforts. These sources give your muscles the energy they need to function and mend.

An example of a muscle-building meal tweak:

Before working exercise, consume a cup of oatmeal with a banana and a scoop of whey protein. To promote muscle growth and repair after a workout, consume grilled salmon with quinoa and steamed veggies.

Improved Overall Health

If your initial goals of increasing muscle mass or decreasing body fat have been met, your nutritional plan will shift to one that emphasizes sustainability and balance, with your current emphasis being to maintain or improve your overall health.

Crucial Changes to Maintain Health:

Macronutrient Balance: Make sure you eat enough fats, proteins, and carbohydrates to meet your maintenance calorie demands. This will allow you to continue your growth while maintaining a consistent level of energy.

Micronutrient Diversification: Variety is not only the spice of life; it is also essential for good health. Incorporate a mix of fruits, veggies, and whole grains into your diet to ensure that you are getting a diverse range of nutrients.

Limit Processed Foods: While occasional indulgences are acceptable, try to reduce your intake of processed foods in favor of whole, nutrient-dense foods that promote longevity and health.

An example of a meal modification for sustaining health:

To increase your consumption of antioxidants and omega-3 fatty acids, make a green smoothie once a day with spinach, kale, berries, and flaxseeds, as well as almond milk.

2. Addendum: Endomorph-Compatible Procedures.

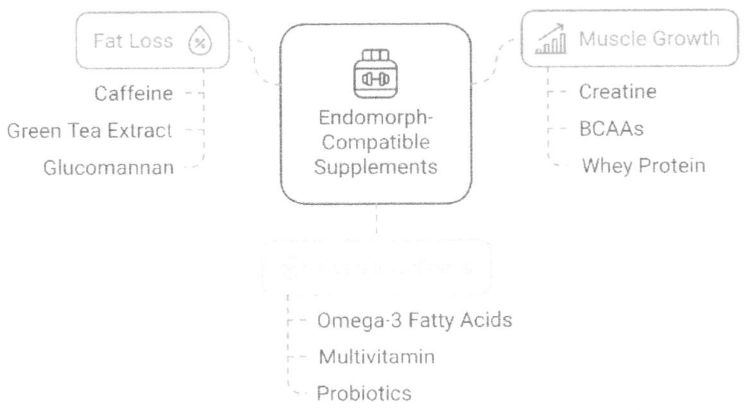

While a well-balanced diet and regular exercise are vital for success, there are various supplements that can help your endomorph body fulfill its specific needs and aid in your goal-achieving process. The idea is to select supplements that are scientifically supported for your specific aims.

Supplements for reducing body fat

Endomorphs may benefit from weight loss supplements that increase metabolism, promote fat burning, and manage blood sugar levels.

Supplements You Should Take to Lose Fat:

Caffeine: is a natural thermogenic that increases fat burning and metabolism, particularly when combined with exercise. Caffeine intake before exercise can boost performance and increase calorie burn.

Green Tea Extract: High in antioxidants, green tea extract has been demonstrated to help reduce body fat by improving the body's ability to burn fat through metabolism.

Glucomannan: By increasing sensations of fullness, this fiber supplement can help manage appetite and reduce cravings, making it simpler to maintain a calorie deficit.

Supplements For Muscle Growth

Endomorphs looking to grow muscle can benefit from supplements that speed up recovery, increase protein synthesis, and boost training performance.

Important Supplements to Gain Muscle:

Creatine is one of the most researched muscle building supplements; it boosts power and strength, allowing you to lift bigger weights and gain muscle faster.

Branch-Chain Amino Acids (BCAAs): Including BCAAs in your post-workout regimen will help lessen soreness and promote recovery.

Whey Protein: Whey protein drinks are quick to digest and high in important amino acids required for muscle growth and repair. They can speed up recovery and promote muscle growth after a workout.

Supplements to Promote Overall Wellness

Endomorphs may concentrate on nutrients that promote good digestion, the immune system, and overall metabolic performance.

Essential Vitamins for Overall Health:

Omega-3 Fatty Acids: These beneficial fats are especially crucial for endomorphs, who may be more prone to metabolic disorders. They also reduce inflammation, strengthen the heart, and improve cognitive functioning.

Multivitamin: A high-quality multivitamin can ensure that you get all of the vital vitamins and minerals you need for good health, as well as assist address nutritional gaps in your diet.

Probiotics: Probiotics improve digestion and gut health, which are necessary for nutrition absorption and overall health.

3. Adjusting Your Exercise Program

Your workout plan is critical to reaching your goals, whether they are to lose fat, gain muscle, or maintain overall fitness. Changing your workouts as you go will ensure that you keep pushing your body and making steady development.

Progressive Overload of Power

Endomorphs are frequently adept at developing muscle and strength. To continue improving in this area, focus on the concept of progressive overload, which involves gradually increasing the weight, repetitions, or intensity of your workouts.

Application of Progressive Overload:

Weight Gain: If you've been lifting the same amount of weight for a while, it's time to increase it. Aim for a 5-10% weight rise every several weeks.

Reps: If you can't increase the weight, try raising the number of repetitions in each set; even a little increase of one or two reps each set can give your muscles a new challenge.

Change the cadence of your lifts to provide a new stimulus for growth. To maximize the amount of time under stress, slow down the eccentric (falling) phase of your lifts.

High-Intensity Interval Training (HIIT): A Method to Reduce Body Fat

High-intensity interval training (HIIT) is one of the best cardio strategies for fat reduction, even for endomorphs who may struggle with traditional steady-state cardio exercises. By including HIIT workouts into your routine, you can burn fat while maintaining muscular mass.

An example of an HIIT workout:

5 minutes of easy running or cycling for a warm-up

30 seconds of maximum effort sprinting, followed by one minute of walking or brisk running.

Continue for eight or ten rounds.

Cool down with five minutes of stretching and light running.

Restorative and Adaptable

Recovery is an important part of your progress as an endomorph; scheduling active recovery, flexibility training, and rest days ensures that your muscles have enough time to develop and repair without causing harm.

Significant Healing Methods:

Stretching and Mobility: After your workout, spend ten to fifteen minutes stretching and doing mobility exercises.

Active Recovery Days: Instead of taking entire rest days, consider including active recovery routines such as yoga, swimming, and walking. These will allow you to keep active without putting undue stress on your body.

Aim for 7 to 9 hours of quality sleep: each night to help you achieve your fitness goals. Sleep is vital for muscle recovery and fat loss.

By implementing these cutting-edge tactics, you will set yourself up for long-term success. Whether you're aiming for fat loss, muscle gain, or overall health with your nutrition, choosing the correct supplements, or fine-tuning your workouts, these simple changes can make a significant difference. Remember that progress is not always linear, but with consistent effort and careful preparation, you may continue to achieve your goals and realize your body's potential. You're only getting started with your makeover, so keep going and stay focused!

Notes

Notes

(Chapter 5:)

Maintaining Your Results.

Achieving your fitness objectives is excellent, but keeping up your progress might be the most difficult part of the process. Developing the mental shift required to move from weight loss to maintenance can help you create long-term, sustainable behaviors. This chapter will walk you through this key phase, focusing on how to make the transition smoothly, form lasting habits, and adopt lifestyle adjustments that enhance long-term health.

1. Making the Switch from Loss to Maintenance of Weight

It's time to shift gears after weeks or months of concentrated weight loss. The move from active weight reduction to maintenance may appear overwhelming, but it does not have to be. The idea is to reset your lifestyle and diet so that you can continue to succeed without having to adhere to the same stringent calorie deficits or tough exercise schedules.

Adjusting Your Calorie Intake

Once you've met your weight-loss target, your body no longer need the same calorie deficit that it did for fat loss. Nonetheless, opting for a steady increase in daily caloric consumption will help you avoid undesirable weight gain.

How to Determine Your Calorie Requirements for Maintenance:

To begin, use one of the many online calculators to calculate your Total Daily Energy Expenditure (TDEE), which is the total number of calories burned by your body during the day.

After calculating your TDEE, gradually increase your weekly caloric intake by 100-200 calories until you reach a maintenance level that feels manageable and prevents fat accumulation.

It is critical to keep an eye on your body as you make these changes. Pay close attention to how you feel, how your clothes fit, and any changes in body composition. If you observe any significant changes, make the appropriate adjustments to keep your body balanced.

Maintaining Muscle Mass

You don't want to lose the muscle you've worked so hard to build when you go into maintenance. Endomorphs require muscular mass to regulate their metabolism and promote long-term fat loss.

Important Techniques for Maintaining Muscle Mass:

Strength Training: If you are no longer in an aggressive fat-loss phase, integrate strength training at least three or four times per week. This will keep your muscles engaged and prevent fat rebound.

Sufficient Protein Consumption: To maintain muscle mass and assist recovery, consume at least 1 gram of protein per pound of body weight, even if you consume more calories.

Prioritize Recovery: Recovery is essential for the long-term maintenance of muscle and overall health. Give your muscles the time they need to regenerate and heal by prioritizing rest and sleep.

Controlling Emotional Change

Achieving your weight-loss target is a significant accomplishment, but it frequently triggers unexpected emotions; some may feel confused or lost because they are no longer actively pursuing fat loss, while others may be concerned that they may regain the weight.

How to Handle Emotional Shifts:

Create New Goals: Once you've met your weight-loss goal, set new goals to keep you motivated. These goals do not have to be about losing weight; they could be about gaining muscle, being in better shape, or even starting a new activity.

Respect Your Achievements: Take a time to reflect on your progress. Respect your accomplishments, and remember that upkeep is just as important as the first adjustment.

Develop Self-Compassion: You are not required to sustain your success by being perfect every day. Life will have ups and downs; therefore, you should be prepared to deal with these events by practicing self-compassion strategies. If you do depart from your regimen, it is critical that you get back on track and continue to grow.

2. Creating Stable Routines

Creating routines that are simple to adopt into your everyday activities is critical for long-term success. These routines should boost your overall physical and mental health. One of the most beneficial aspects of developing habits is that they gradually become second nature, making it simpler to continue your success without continuously feeling like you're "on a diet."

Creating Effective Routines

Behavior stacking refers to the process of merging a new behavior with an existing one. It's one of the most effective strategies to form new habits since it makes it easy to include into your daily routine and promotes consistency.

The examples of habit stacking are as follows:

Morning Hydration: If you already brew coffee in the morning, make it a habit to drink a glass of water first thing. This will help you keep hydrated and increase your metabolism.

Pre-gym Routine: If you exercise at a certain time of day, make it a habit to lay out your gym clothes the night before. This allows you to mentally prepare for the activity at hand and eliminates any distractions that might cause you to miss your session.

Walking after dinner aids digestion and keeps you in shape. If you usually watch TV after dinner, go for a 10-minute stroll before or after.

Consistency takes precedence over perfection.

In terms of dependability, consistency trumps perfection. A widespread fallacy is that missing a workout or eating a lavish meal will erase all of your efforts. In actuality, what is most important is your long-term behavior.

Advice to Maintain Consistency:

Prioritize growth Over Perfection: Instead of striving for perfection, set a goal of consistent growth. It's normal to have better weeks than bad weeks as long as your behaviors remain consistent.

Use a Habit Tracker: Tracking your daily actions, such as water consumption and exercise, is an excellent method to hold yourself accountable. You can use either a mobile app or a physical habit tracker.

Include Flexibility in Your Routine: Rigidity leads to tiredness since life is unpredictable. Be adaptable with your routine and habits, allowing yourself to change as circumstances require.

Methods for Mindful Consumption

Mindful eating is one of the most important habits to develop for long-term maintenance. This allows you to learn to trust your body's hunger and fullness cues rather than adhering to strict diet regimens or tracking your caloric intake.

Tips For Mindful Eating:

Eat Slowly: Eating slowly helps you avoid overeating by allowing your body to identify fullness with each bite and giving you time to chew and appreciate it.

Recognize Your Hunger Signals: Before you grab a snack, examine if you're actually hungry or if you're eating out of habit, stress, or boredom.

Enjoy Treats in Moderation: Remember that one indulgence will not ruin all of your hard work, so use them judiciously and guilt-free. Being in the black does not imply giving up on your favorite meals. Moderation is the key.

3. Lifestyle Changes for Long-term Health

In addition to diet and exercise, keeping your results entails leading a lifestyle that supports long-term health and fitness rather than just weight loss. This involves stress management, appropriate sleep, and the development of strong support systems.

Prioritizing sleep for recovery and overall well-being.

Sleep is one of the most critical, yet frequently disregarded, parts of long-term health. Inadequate sleep can cause stress, weight gain, difficulties sustaining results, hormone imbalance, muscle repair issues, and poor mental and physical health.

Tips For Getting the Best Sleep for Recovery:

Create a Sleep Plan: You can improve the quality of your sleep and support your body's internal clock by following a regular sleep schedule that includes going to bed and waking up at the same times every day.

Limit Your Pre-Bed Screen Time: Computers, phones, and tablets emit blue light, which can interfere with your body's melatonin production, making it more difficult to fall asleep. Aim for at least 30 minutes of screen-free time before bedtime.

Create a serene environment: Your bedroom should be a quiet, dark, and cool area to unwind.

You should also purchase a comfy mattress and pillows to support healthy sleep.

Stress Reduction for Long-Term Health.

Chronic stress can harm your health and hinder your ability to lose weight. Hormone imbalances, sleeplessness, and emotional eating are just a few of the drawbacks that can stall your development. Stress management is critical for maintaining peak performance and general well-being.

Realistic Stress Reduction Techniques:

Mindfulness Meditation: Practicing mindfulness and meditation every day, even for five to ten minutes, can help you stay present, reduce stress, and enhance your mental health.

Exercise for Stress Reduction: Physical activity can help people manage their weight and reduce stress. Yoga, walking, and dancing are examples of endorphin-releasing and stress-relieving activities that you can add into your daily routine.

Writing down your thoughts and feelings might help you control your emotions and deal with stress. By analyzing your journal entries, you can spot any stress-related trends that need to be addressed.

Developing a Network of Assistance

Being surrounded by people who support you to maintain your healthy habits can have a big impact on your long-term health and weight loss goals.

How to build a valuable network:

Find Accountability Partners: Find someone who shares your health goals or who exercises alongside you. Having someone hold you accountable helps you stay motivated and motivates you to stick to your program.

Join a community: Connecting with like-minded people in a local gym class, social media group, or online forum can provide encouragement, support, and guidance.

Involve Your Friends and Family: Discuss your health goals with your loved ones and include them in your journey. Your inner circle's support is vital, whether you're preparing healthy meals or embarking on challenging trips.

Notes

Notes

(Chapter 6:)

Clarifications and Questions.

It's normal to have concerns while you work toward your health and fitness goals, especially if you identify as an endomorph. There is a lot of misinformation out there, and it can be tough to separate fact from fantasy. This chapter answers the most typical questions that emerge when following the endomorph eating plan, with the purpose of removing any misunderstanding and giving you the confidence to move on, knowing that you have the resources you need to succeed.

1. Frequently Asked Questions.

Are endomorphs truly slower at losing weight than other body types?

Individuals with an endomorph body type frequently complain that losing weight is more difficult and time-consuming. This is somewhat correct, as endomorphs often have slower metabolisms, making it easier to accumulate fat and more difficult to shed it. This is not to say that endomorphs cannot lose weight; with a specialized diet, continuous exercise, and prudent lifestyle modifications, they can accomplish significant fat loss. Understanding how your body works and adhering to a long-term plan are more vital than seeking quick fixes.

I am an endomorph; is it okay for me to eat carbohydrates?

A: Carbohydrates are fine. Endomorphs are more sensitive to insulin spikes and carbohydrates; thus, the timing and kind of carbs are critical. Choose complex carbs over simple carbohydrates, such as those found in vegetables, whole grains, and legumes, because they release energy gradually and do not raise blood sugar levels. It's also vital to organize your carb consumption around your workouts because your body uses carbohydrates for fuel and muscle repair most efficiently while exercising. In general, you should strive for a diet heavy in protein and moderate in fat, with the majority of your carbohydrates coming early in the day or right before your workouts.

Which sort of exercise should I emphasize, strength training or cardio?

A: Endomorphs should not underestimate the value of strength training, even though cardio is frequently seen as the most effective approach to reduce weight. Weightlifting builds muscle, which raises metabolism and promotes more effective fat loss. To get the best results, combine cardio and weight training. Strength training should be the foundation of your approach, with cardio (such as steady-state cardio or HIIT) helping to expedite fat loss. In summary, aim to lift weights three to four times a week and incorporate aerobic exercises as needed.

MEGAN

How much protein is recommended per day?

A: Each meal should include high-quality protein sources such as fish, eggs, lean meats, Greek yogurt, and plant-based meals like beans and legumes. Endomorphs require even more protein, so aim for 1.1-1.2 grams per pound of body weight to maintain muscle mass while decreasing fat and increasing muscle growth and recovery. Furthermore, protein increases sensations of fullness, allowing you to fight cravings and overindulge.

What should I do if my weight loss efforts aren't progressing?

A: Hitting a plateau is a common part of any weight-loss journey, and while it can be discouraging, it usually indicates that your body has adapted to your routine and requires some changes.

Here are some ideas to assist you overcome a plateau:

Adjust your calorie intake: If you've been in a calorie deficit for a while, your body may have altered how it uses energy. To assist your metabolism reset, consider eating a little more at first, then gradually decrease it.

Mix up your workouts: Make your sessions more challenging by using heavier weights, more repetitions, or various exercises that put your body through new challenges.

Add High-Intensity Interval Training (HIIT): This efficient fat-burning strategy does not necessitate long treadmill sessions; instead, it consists of short bursts of intense exercise alternated with rest intervals to shake your body out of a plateau.

Get more sleep: When you reach a plateau, your body may require additional time to repair. Make sure you get enough sleep and take rest days so your body can rebuild and regenerate.

Is intermittent fasting an effective technique for endomorphs?

A: Intermittent fasting (IF) is an effective method for endomorphs who struggle with portion sizes and calorie intake. By reducing you're eating window, you may automatically minimize the number of meals and snacks you consume, allowing you to better control your calorie intake and promote weight loss. However, not everyone is suitable for IF. If you discover that fasting causes you to overeat later in the day or lowers your energy levels, it may not be the best strategy for you. The most important thing is to develop a long-term, sustainable eating plan.

How can I avoid gaining weight again once I've attained my goal?

A: Preventing weight gain is a major issue, particularly for endomorphs who believe their bodies were designed to gain weight swiftly. The key to retaining your results is consistency and long-term habit building. You must transition from a caloric deficit to maintenance calories, remembering to gradually increase your intake while prioritizing high-fiber carbs, healthy fats, and protein. To maintain muscle mass and a healthy metabolism, you must continue to strength train and participate in physical exercise. Keep an eye on your progress and change your behaviors if you notice any unnecessary weight returning.

2. Debunking Endomorph Myths

There are numerous myths surrounding fitness and diets, and regrettably, endomorphs are frequently misinformed about factors that may impede their development. Let's discuss and clear up some of the most common misconceptions concerning endomorphs.

Myth 1: Endomorphs are "doomed" to obesity.

Truth: Being an endomorph does not imply fat. Although endomorphs are more likely to accumulate fat, it is still feasible to acquire a lean, healthy figure by building muscle and decreasing weight. The goal is to understand your specific metabolic tendencies and tailor your food, exercise routine, and lifestyle to them. If you are motivated and take the necessary procedures, you may disprove this misconception and get long-term results.

Myth 2: Endomorphs should avoid carbs completely.

Truth: This is a frequent myth. While endomorphs should limit their carbohydrate intake, eliminating them completely is not necessary—in fact, it may have the opposite effect. Carbohydrates are a crucial source of energy, particularly for people who exercise on a daily basis. The answer is to eat the appropriate carbs, specifically complex, slow-digesting carbs that provide long-term energy without raising blood sugar levels.

Myth 3: Endomorphs need to exercise for hours on end to lose weight.

Truth: While exercise might aid in fat loss, it is a fallacy that endomorphs must run continually to achieve results. The most effective strategy to grow muscle and burn fat is to combine moderate cardio with strength training. Endomorphs require muscular mass since it boosts metabolism and promotes fat loss. Instead of spending hours on the treadmill, concentrate on muscle development through strength training and effective cardio such as HIIT.

Myth 4: Endomorphs will always acquire weight, regardless of their behavior.

Truth: Although endomorphs are more likely to acquire weight, this does not imply that you will uncontrollably regain all of the weight you lose.

You can permanently lose weight by eating a good diet, exercising, and living a balanced lifestyle. Gaining muscle mass is especially important for long-term weight management since it boosts metabolism. You can keep on track by tracking your progress and making minor changes to your diet and exercise regimen.

Myth 5: Endomorphs respond well to a specific diet.

Truth: Success depends on individuality and flexibility. Even people with comparable body types exhibit varying physical traits. Endomorphs cannot adhere to a one-size-fits-all diet and activity plan; what works for one individual may not work for another. The best course of action is to experiment with different strategies to see what works best for your body, such as adjusting macronutrient ratios, meal time, or exercise routines.

Myth 6: Endomorphs require less food to maintain their current weight.

Truth: Limiting your consumption is not always the greatest strategy to manage your weight, especially for endomorphs. Instead, focus on eating more intelligently and prioritizing nutrient-dense foods that keep you full and provide long-lasting energy. Restricting your intake makes it more difficult to maintain your weight because your metabolism slows down if you're constantly starving yourself. Regular exercise, combined with a well-balanced diet high in protein, healthy fats, and complex carbohydrates, will help you keep your results without feeling cheated or weary.

To summarize, let us congratulate your accomplishments and go beyond the diet.

As you look ahead, keep in mind that this journey requires much more than simply following a diet; you've already accomplished a lot by reaching this final chapter. You've taken the time to discover, comprehend, and implement a method tailored to your body type. You now have the knowledge to change your lifestyle while also achieving your weight loss goals. There have been setbacks along the way, but each one has helped you undergo significant internal transformations.

Recognize Your Success

Take a moment to reflect on your progress. No matter how far along you are or how many major changes you have already gone through, each step of this journey deserves to be celebrated. Fitness and weight loss are about more than just achieving a certain weight or looking good. They are about the small and large victories you have achieved through your own hard work and dedication.

Individual Victories:

More Than Just Physiological Changes

It is easy to become obsessed with the physical signs of weight loss, such as a smaller waist circumference and a more toned physique. However, these superficial changes are not the only factors influencing your success. Consider the mental and emotional transformation you've undergone. Perhaps you feel more confident in yourself, have more energy throughout the day, or have improved your self-discipline and control.

These intangible victories are equally, if not more important, than tangible ones. They represent a deeper shift within you: you are becoming more resilient, capable of overcoming obstacles, and aware of your body's needs. You won't need a "diet" to reap the benefits of these skills; they will shape your attitudes toward food, fitness, and self-care for the rest of your life.

Tracking Development: Recognize Minor Wins.

When you think back on your trip, it's important to celebrate your small wins as well as your big ones. Did you set a new personal record in the gym? Celebrate it! Did you stick to your diet and avoid temptations for the entire week? That's amazing!

Did you overcome a setback and continue pursuing your objectives? Celebrate that persistence.

By celebrating these small wins, you may reinforce the positive changes you're making. You change your mindset from one of powerlessness or hardship to one of empowerment and pride. Each small win is a reminder of your commitment and development.

Building Self-Belief: The Power of Success

Success multiplies like wildfire. As you celebrate more victories, you'll feel more confident that you can keep up a healthy lifestyle. You need this confidence to sustain your results over time. It reminds you that you can overcome challenges even when things get tough. Motivation comes from confidence, and motivation keeps you moving forward.

So go ahead and celebrate yourself. You deserve it. Whether it's with a nice dinner, a new gym outfit, or just by looking back at how far you've come, take a moment to acknowledge your efforts.

The Journey Other Than the Diet

Once you've achieved your initial weight-loss goals, it's imperative that you shift your mindset from one of a short-term diet to one of a long-term lifestyle strategy. The progress you've made thanks to this program is just getting started; in order to maintain and even improve your results, you need to acknowledge that wellness and health are journeys rather than destination.

MEGAN

Sustainability as opposed to Perfection

One of the biggest challenges people face after reaching their goals is fear of "falling off the wagon" or gaining back the weight they have worked so hard to lose. This fear can lead to an all-or-nothing mindset, where you feel you have to be perfect to maintain your results, even though perfection is neither necessary nor sustainable.

Choose balance over perfection as your goal. There will always be times in life when you have to stray from your plan, whether it's for a family get-together, vacation, or just a bad day. These occurrences are typical and don't sum up your achievement. It matters what you do with them. Instead of dwelling on guilt or giving up, make an effort to return to your original course as soon as you can. Long-term outcomes are the consequence of consistency over time rather than momentary excellence.

Creating a Lifestyle That Suits You

You don't have to give up all luxuries or adhere to a strict routine for the rest of your life; in fact, trying to do so may make you feel tired and hostile toward the very routines you're trying to maintain. Instead, the key to maintaining your success going forward is creating a lifestyle that suits you. This involves finding a balance between your enjoyable activities and healthy routines.

Instead, focus on creating a flexible plan that allows for both enjoyment and discipline. Examples of this could be giving yourself permission to take days off when your body requires them, allowing yourself to occasionally indulge in your favorite foods, or experimenting with different fitness regimens that keep you inspired and engaged. The goal is to create a routine that is enjoyable, sustainable, and consistent with your long-term health goals.

The Strength of Habits: Establishing a Firm Basis

The foundation of your new way of life is likely a number of routines you've developed along the way that have helped you succeed, such as meal planning, regular exercise, or mindfulness training. The more you support these habits, the more automatic they become and eventually require less conscious effort on your part and just become part of your daily routine.

But remember that habits take time to form, and it's normal to experience moments when forming new habits feels hard or when old habits start to resurface. The key is to persevere through the process, even if it is difficult at times, because daily practice of these behaviors strengthens your foundation for long-term success.

The Benefits of Lifelong Learning

The knowledge you have gained thus far is not the end of your journey beyond the diet. The fields of fitness, nutrition, and wellness are dynamic; remaining current will help you continue to make the healthiest decisions for your body. As you proceed, be open-minded, experiment with different strategies, and seek out new information to determine what works best for you.

Whether it's finding new recipes that fit your goals, learning more about advanced training techniques, or figuring out how to get the most out of your sleep and recovery, ongoing education is crucial to keeping interest and motivation high. Be open to changing as your body and needs do.

Lifestyle Changes for Long-Term Health

While your initial reason for being on this journey was to lose weight, you've realized that health is much more than a number on a scale. Put your overall wellness first as you transition from a weight-loss attitude to one that is focused on your long-term health.

Stress the Application of Functional Fitness

As you continue to exercise, move your attention from simply cosmetic aims to functional fitness, which is teaching your body to perform well during everyday tasks like lifting, running, stretching, or just moving around with ease. Functional fitness increases your life quality, minimizes the chance of injury, and ensures that you will be able to enjoy physical activities for a very long time.

Give stress management and mental wellness a priority.

Mental wellness is a crucial component of overall wellness, while being often overlooked in the pursuit of physical fitness. Effective coping mechanisms for long-term stress are crucial since they can have adverse consequences on your weight, metabolism, and overall well-being.

Prioritize your mental health, whether it is through journaling, meditation, time spent in nature, or engaging in your favorite pastimes. Your body is more likely to behave properly when your mind is well.

Acknowledge the importance of lifelong learning and growth.

Finally, remember that health and wellness are dynamic ideas. As you grow and evolve, so will your needs, ambitions, and difficulties. Embrace the reality that you will have opportunity to learn, grow, and discover who you are throughout your life as you walk this road.

You may fully utilize your body's potential and design a vibrant, meaningful existence that is in line with your highest goals if you invest more time in yourself.

Final Words

As you move forward, remember that sustaining your health is a lifetime endeavor that takes self-compassion, adaptability, and patience. You've come a long way, and your accomplishments are a result of your perseverance, commitment, and readiness to accept change.

Respect your success, but do not stop there. Continue on this journey and let it shape not only your appearance but also your overall personality. You still have your finest days ahead of you, and you can accomplish everything you put your mind to.

What more could you want than a life filled with achievement, joy, and health?

Thank you for reading!

I'd like to personally thank you for taking the time to read my work. I really appreciate your time and effort, and I hope this book has provided you with valuable success tools and insights.

Your feedback is really useful to me as I grow as a writer. I would love to hear your feedback, whether positive or negative, so that I may develop and make future works even more useful and fascinating.

I humbly request that you offer an honest review if you found this book worthwhile or if you believe anything may be improved. Your counsel will help me not only improve, but also become a better person.

Thank you again for your support, and I look forward to hearing from you!

SINCERLY

MEGAN

Notes

Notes

Weekly Measurements Tracker

Week	Arms	Chest	Waist	Hips	Thigh
Week 01					
Week 02					
Week 03					
Week 04					
Week 05					
Week 06					
Week 07					
Week 08					
Week 09					
Week 10					
Week 11					
Week 12					
Week 13					
Week 14					
Week 15					
Week 16					
Week 17					
Week 18					
Week 19					
Week 20					
Week 21					
Week 22					
Week 23					
Week 24					
Week 25					
Week 26					
Week 27					
Week 28					
Week 29					

MEGAN

Weekly Measurements Tracker

Week	Arms	Chest	Waist	Hips	Thigh
Week 30					
Week 31					
Week 32					
Week 33					
Week 34					
Week 35					
Week 36					
Week 37					
Week 38					
Week 39					
Week 40					
Week 41					
Week 42					
Week 43					
Week 44					
Week 45					
Week 46					
Week 47					
Week 48					
Week 49					
Week 50					
Week 51					
Week 52					

Weekly Measurements Tracker

Week	Arms	Chest	Waist	Hips	Thigh
Week 01					
Week 02					
Week 03					
Week 04					
Week 05					
Week 06					
Week 07					
Week 08					
Week 09					
Week 10					
Week 11					
Week 12					
Week 13					
Week 14					
Week 15					
Week 16					
Week 17					
Week 18					
Week 19					
Week 20					
Week 21					
Week 22					
Week 23					
Week 24					
Week 25					
Week 26					
Week 27					
Week 28					
Week 29					

MEGAN

Weekly Measurements Tracker

Week	Arms	Chest	Waist	Hips	Thigh
Week 30					
Week 31					
Week 32					
Week 33					
Week 34					
Week 35					
Week 36					
Week 37					
Week 38					
Week 39					
Week 40					
Week 41					
Week 42					
Week 43					
Week 44					
Week 45					
Week 46					
Week 47					
Week 48					
Week 49					
Week 50					
Week 51					
Week 52					

Weekly Measurements Tracker

Week	Arms	Chest	Waist	Hips	Thigh
Week 01					
Week 02					
Week 03					
Week 04					
Week 05					
Week 06					
Week 07					
Week 08					
Week 09					
Week 10					
Week 11					
Week 12					
Week 13					
Week 14					
Week 15					
Week 16					
Week 17					
Week 18					
Week 19					
Week 20					
Week 21					
Week 22					
Week 23					
Week 24					
Week 25					
Week 26					
Week 27					
Week 28					
Week 29					

MEGAN

Weekly Measurements Tracker

Week	Arms	Chest	Waist	Hips	Thigh
Week 30					
Week 31					
Week 32					
Week 33					
Week 34					
Week 35					
Week 36					
Week 37					
Week 38					
Week 39					
Week 40					
Week 41					
Week 42					
Week 43					
Week 44					
Week 45					
Week 46					
Week 47					
Week 48					
Week 49					
Week 50					
Week 51					
Week 52					

Weekly Measurements Tracker

Week	Arms	Chest	Waist	Hips	Thigh
Week 01					
Week 02					
Week 03					
Week 04					
Week 05					
Week 06					
Week 07					
Week 08					
Week 09					
Week 10					
Week 11					
Week 12					
Week 13					
Week 14					
Week 15					
Week 16					
Week 17					
Week 18					
Week 19					
Week 20					
Week 21					
Week 22					
Week 23					
Week 24					
Week 25					
Week 26					
Week 27					
Week 28					
Week 29					

MEGAN

Weekly Measurements Tracker

Week	Arms	Chest	Waist	Hips	Thigh
Week 30					
Week 31					
Week 32					
Week 33					
Week 34					
Week 35					
Week 36					
Week 37					
Week 38					
Week 39					
Week 40					
Week 41					
Week 42					
Week 43					
Week 44					
Week 45					
Week 46					
Week 47					
Week 48					
Week 49					
Week 50					
Week 51					
Week 52					

Habit Tracker

Week:

Habit	Sun	Mon	Tue	Wed	Thu	Fri	Sat

MEGAN

Habit Tracker

Week:

Habit	Sun	Mon	Tue	Wed	Thu	Fri	Sat

Habit Tracker

Week:

Habit	Sun	Mon	Tue	Wed	Thu	Fri	Sat

MEGAN

Habit Tracker

Week:

Habit	Sun	Mon	Tue	Wed	Thu	Fri	Sat

Weekly Meal Planner

	Breakfast	Lunch	Snack	Dinner
Monday				
Tuesday				
Wednesday				
Thursday				
Friday				
Saturday				
Sunday				

Notes

MEGAN

Weekly Meal Planner

	Breakfast	Lunch	Snack	Dinner
Monday				
Tuesday				
Wednesday				
Thursday				
Friday				
Saturday				
Sunday				

Notes

Weekly Meal Planner

	Breakfast	Lunch	Snack	Dinner
Monday				
	Breakfast	Lunch	Snack	Dinner
Tuesday				
	Breakfast	Lunch	Snack	Dinner
Wednesday				
	Breakfast	Lunch	Snack	Dinner
Thursday				
	Breakfast	Lunch	Snack	Dinner
Friday				
	Breakfast	Lunch	Snack	Dinner
Saturday				
	Breakfast	Lunch	Snack	Dinner
Sunday				

Notes

MEGAN

Weekly Meal Planner

	Breakfast	Lunch	Snack	Dinner
Monday				
Tuesday				
Wednesday				
Thursday				
Friday				
Saturday				
Sunday				

Notes

Weekly Workout Tracker

Week Of:

Monday

Tuesday

Wednesday

Thursday

Friday

Saturday

Sunday

Calories Burned

Monday	Friday
Tuesday	Saturday
Wednesday	Sunday
Thursday	Total:

MEGAN

Weekly Workout Tracker

Week Of:

Monday	Tuesday	Wednesday

Thursday	Friday	Saturday

Sunday

Calories Burned

Monday	Friday
Tuesday	Saturday
Wednesday	Sunday
Thursday	Total:

Weekly Workout Tracker

Week Of:

Monday

Tuesday

Wednesday

Thursday

Friday

Saturday

Sunday

Calories Burned

Monday	Friday
Tuesday	Saturday
Wednesday	Sunday
Thursday	Total:

MEGAN

Weekly Workout Tracker

Week Of:

Monday	Tuesday	Wednesday

Thursday	Friday	Saturday

Sunday

Calories Burned

Monday	Friday
Tuesday	Saturday
Wednesday	Sunday
Thursday	Total:

Food Tracker

	Breakfast	Lunch	Dinner
Monday			
	Breakfast	Lunch	Dinner
Tuesday			
	Breakfast	Lunch	Dinner
Wednesday			
	Breakfast	Lunch	Dinner
Thursday			
	Breakfast	Lunch	Dinner
Friday			
	Breakfast	Lunch	Dinner
Saturday			
	Breakfast	Lunch	Dinner
Sunday			

MEGAN

Food Tracker

	Breakfast	Lunch	Dinner
Monday			
	Breakfast	Lunch	Dinner
Tuesday			
	Breakfast	Lunch	Dinner
Wednesday			
	Breakfast	Lunch	Dinner
Thursday			
	Breakfast	Lunch	Dinner
Friday			
	Breakfast	Lunch	Dinner
Saturday			
	Breakfast	Lunch	Dinner
Sunday			

Food Tracker

	Breakfast	Lunch	Dinner
Monday			
Tuesday			
Wednesday			
Thursday			
Friday			
Saturday			
Sunday			

Food Tracker

Monday	Breakfast	Lunch	Dinner

Tuesday	Breakfast	Lunch	Dinner

Wednesday	Breakfast	Lunch	Dinner

Thursday	Breakfast	Lunch	Dinner

Friday	Breakfast	Lunch	Dinner

Saturday	Breakfast	Lunch	Dinner

Sunday	Breakfast	Lunch	Dinner

Favorite Foods Tracker

Food	Fat	Protein	Carbs	Sugars	Calories

MEGAN

Favorite Foods Tracker

Food	Fat	Protein	Carbs	Sugars	Calories

Favorite Foods Tracker

Food	Fat	Protein	Carbs	Sugars	Calories

MEGAN

Favorite Foods Tracker

Food	Fat	Protein	Carbs	Sugars	Calories

Workout Log

Date	Activity	Energy	Time	Sets	Reps	Dist.	Wgt.

MEGAN

Workout Log

Date	Activity	Energy	Time	Sets	Reps	Dist.	Wgt.

Workout Log

Date	Activity	Energy	Time	Sets	Reps	Dist.	Wgt.

MEGAN

Workout Log

Date	Activity	Energy	Time	Sets	Reps	Dist.	Wgt.

Sleep Tracker

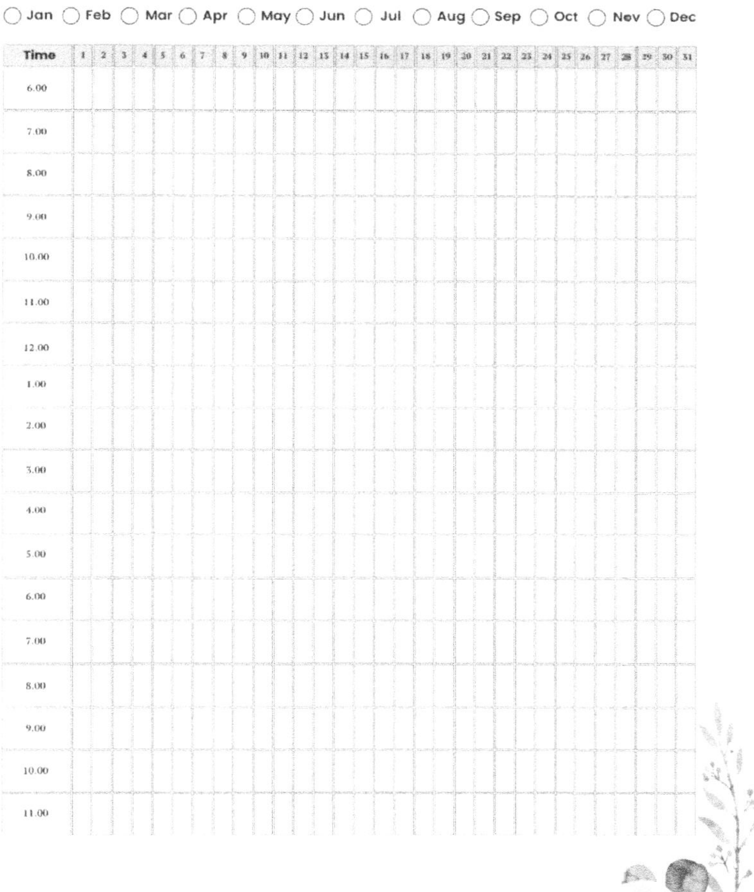

◯ Jan ◯ Feb ◯ Mar ◯ Apr ◯ May ◯ Jun ◯ Jul ◯ Aug ◯ Sep ◯ Oct ◯ Nov ◯ Dec

Time	1	2	3	4	5	6	7	8	9	10	11	12	13	14	15	16	17	18	19	20	21	22	23	24	25	26	27	28	29	30	31
6.00																															
7.00																															
8.00																															
9.00																															
10.00																															
11.00																															
12.00																															
1.00																															
2.00																															
3.00																															
4.00																															
5.00																															
6.00																															
7.00																															
8.00																															
9.00																															
10.00																															
11.00																															

Sleep Tracker

◯ Jan ◯ Feb ◯ Mar ◯ Apr ◯ May ◯ Jun ◯ Jul ◯ Aug ◯ Sep ◯ Oct ◯ Nov ◯ Dec

Time	1	2	3	4	5	6	7	8	9	10	11	12	13	14	15	16	17	18	19	20	21	22	23	24	25	26	27	28	29	30	31
6.00																															
7.00																															
8.00																															
9.00																															
10.00																															
11.00																															
12.00																															
1.00																															
2.00																															
3.00																															
4.00																															
5.00																															
6.00																															
7.00																															
8.00																															
9.00																															
10.00																															
11.00																															

Sleep Tracker

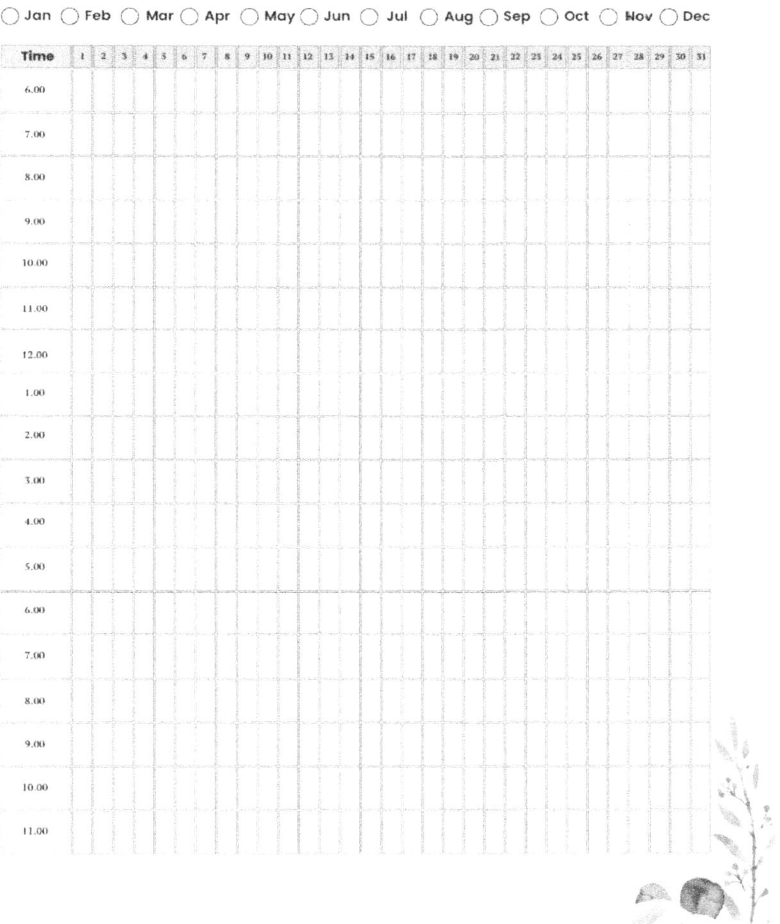

◯ Jan ◯ Feb ◯ Mar ◯ Apr ◯ May ◯ Jun ◯ Jul ◯ Aug ◯ Sep ◯ Oct ◯ Nov ◯ Dec

Time	1	2	3	4	5	6	7	8	9	10	11	12	13	14	15	16	17	18	19	20	21	22	23	24	25	26	27	28	29	30	31
6.00																															
7.00																															
8.00																															
9.00																															
10.00																															
11.00																															
12.00																															
1.00																															
2.00																															
3.00																															
4.00																															
5.00																															
6.00																															
7.00																															
8.00																															
9.00																															
10.00																															
11.00																															

Sleep Tracker

◯ Jan ◯ Feb ◯ Mar ◯ Apr ◯ May ◯ Jun ◯ Jul ◯ Aug ◯ Sep ◯ Oct ◯ Nov ◯ Dec

Time	1	2	3	4	5	6	7	8	9	10	11	12	13	14	15	16	17	18	19	20	21	22	23	24	25	26	27	28	29	30	31
6.00																															
7.00																															
8.00																															
9.00																															
10.00																															
11.00																															
12.00																															
1.00																															
2.00																															
3.00																															
4.00																															
5.00																															
6.00																															
7.00																															
8.00																															
9.00																															
10.00																															
11.00																															

My Daily Fitness

Date: ____________________

My Daily Goals

Exercise Schedule

Type	Reps	Calories

Breakfast

Lunch

Dinner

Water Tracker

Hours To Sleep

MEGAN

My Daily Fitness

Date: ____________________

My Daily Goals

Exercise Schedule

Type	Reps	Calories

Breakfast

Lunch

Dinner

Water Tracker

Hours To Sleep

My Daily Fitness

Date: ____________________

My Daily Goals

____

____

____

____

____

____

____

Exercise Schedule

Type	Reps	Calories

Breakfast

____

____

Lunch

____

____

Dinner

____

____

Water Tracker

Hours To Sleep

MEGAN

My Daily Fitness

Date: ______________

My Daily Goals

Exercise Schedule

Type	Reps	Calories

Breakfast

Lunch

Dinner

Water Tracker

Hours To Sleep

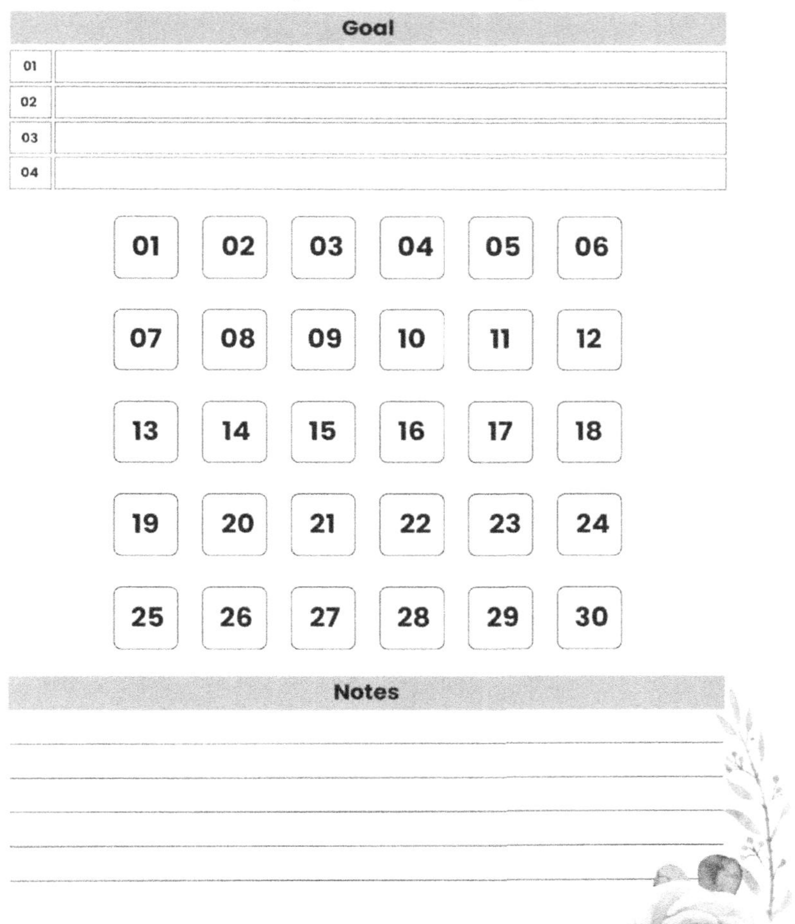

30 Day Challenge

Goal	
01	
02	
03	
04	

01	02	03	04	05	06
07	08	09	10	11	12
13	14	15	16	17	18
19	20	21	22	23	24
25	26	27	28	29	30

Notes

MEGAN

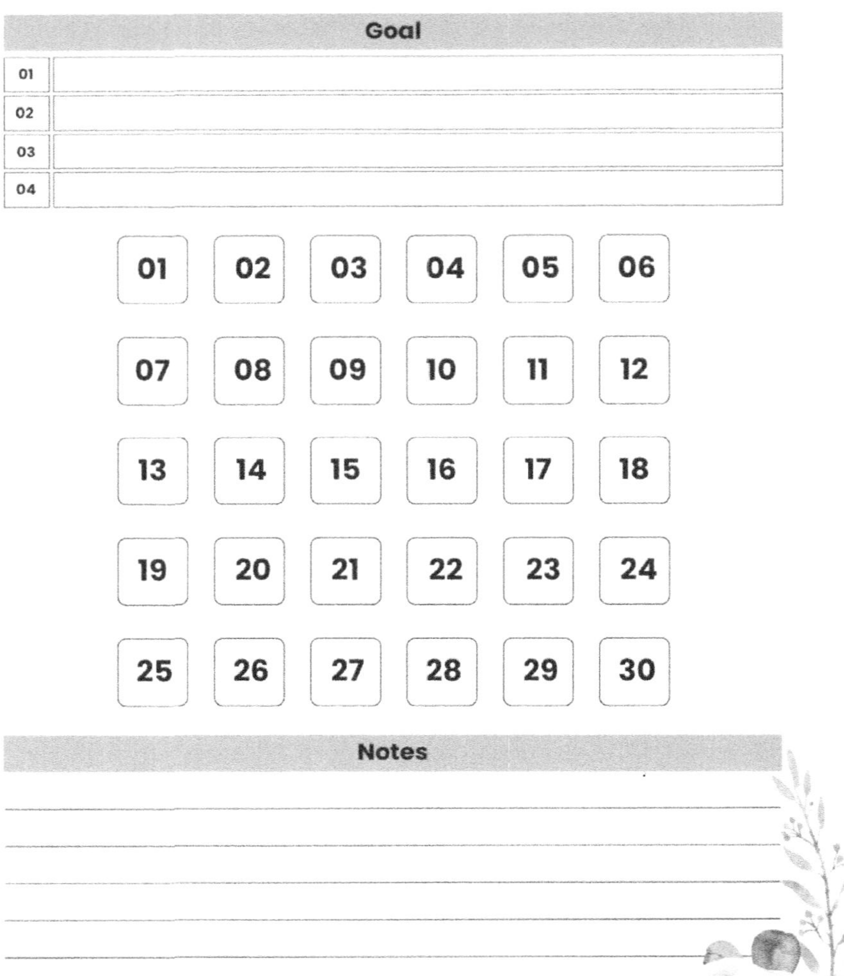

30 Day Challenge

	Goal
01	
02	
03	
04	

01	02	03	04	05	06
07	08	09	10	11	12
13	14	15	16	17	18
19	20	21	22	23	24
25	26	27	28	29	30

Notes

30 Day Challenge

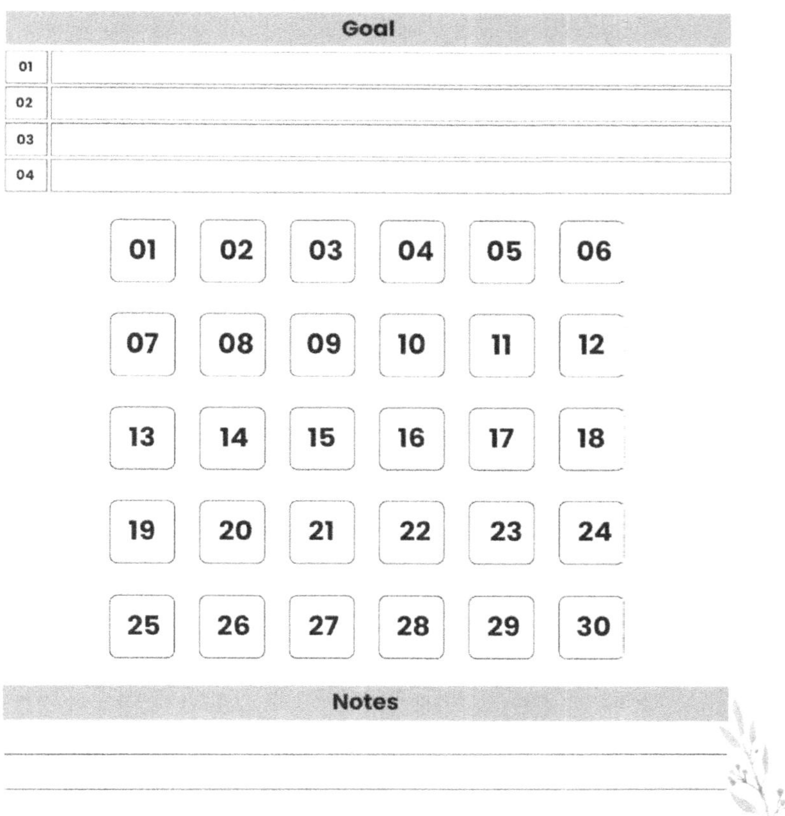

MEGAN

30 Day Challenge

Goal	
01	
02	
03	
04	

01	02	03	04	05	06
07	08	09	10	11	12
13	14	15	16	17	18
19	20	21	22	23	24
25	26	27	28	29	30

Notes

90 Days Body Goals

Goals:	
Reward:	
Start Date:	End Date:

MOTIVATION	ACTION STEPS

NOTES

MEGAN

90 Days Body Goals

Goals:	
Reward:	
Start Date:	End Date:

MOTIVATION	ACTION STEPS

NOTES

90 Days Body Goals

Goals:	
Reward:	
Start Date:	End Date:

MOTIVATION	ACTION STEPS

NOTES

MEGAN

90 Days Body Goals

Goals:	
Reward:	
Start Date:	End Date:

MOTIVATION	ACTION STEPS

NOTES

Made in United States
North Haven, CT
30 March 2025

67370481R00114